Vascular Dementia: The Complete Dementia Caregivers Guide With Tips On Dementia and What You Need to Know to Manage the Condition From the Onset of Dementia Symptoms Today!

By Brian Jeff

~~~

Disclaimer

Table Of Contents

Overview: Dementia and the Screening...

Without doubt the word Dementia is a medical term used to refer to a number of symptoms of cognitive degeneration such as forgetfulness, which moderates a person's ability to perform everyday undertakings.

However, the diagnostic procedure begins with your health practitioner evaluating your medical history as well as that of your parents, siblings, and grandparents.

Yes, I must say here that other possible causes of memory impairment cannot be ruled out. However, a physical examination and blood tests will help eliminate these possibilities.

Besides that, a cognitive test may also be administered in which the patient is asked to perform simple memory processing tasks. The patient may then be referred for more complex medical screenings should the need arise.

As a matter of fact, several types of brain imaging tests, such as CAT scans, MRIs, and PET scans, are usually used to rule out strokes or tumors. The truth is that Dementia can also be caused by a series of strokes so small as to be undetected.

Moreover, it is also known that Depression can equally cause memory lapses. Yes, among many others, Parkinson's disease, a degenerative nerve disorder, can also be a cause of dementia.

Besides, some medications, especially in older patients, can cause fuzzy thinking and memory loss. Even a fever or a head injury can result in memory problems, as can dehydration or malnutrition. Late-stage syphilis is yet another cause of dementia.

However, with blood tests, the practitioners can help eliminate these and other possible causes of memory loss, such as thyroid disorders or vitamin deficiencies.

To be thorough, more extensive neuropsychological testing may be performed on the patient. These tests evaluate the patient's memory, problem-solving abilities, attention span and skills involving numbers and language.

Yes, as a matter of fact, Psychological tests can also be useful in diagnosing Alzheimer's disease.

To further help, a vaccine was developed that reduces the deposits in the brain associated with dementia. However, it was found to have dangerous side effect so, the clinical trial was abandoned.

Though, genetic testing for Alzheimer's disease is still in the beginning phase, nevertheless, researchers have identified several genes that are related to Alzheimer's disease.

It must, however, be stated here that recent studies have shown that only 30% of cognitive decline is the result of genetics. The remaining 70% is the result of lifestyle choices.

So, with what science knows now, the fact is that dementia disease is not a normal part of the human aging process. Yes, there is always a cause, and we have enumerated them above!

Be that as it may, the truth is that physicians have no definitive tests for Alzheimer's disease currently; however, you should not ignore any early symptoms of mental decline.

Without a doubt, there is a new ten-minute test which determines whether a person has dementia… this test is referred to as the paired associates learning (PAL) test.

This has opened the door of possibilities for dementia treatment, and this can also open many doors for new drugs, which may be diagnosed on the live subject.

Yes, with this test, the doctors can now make a distinction between dementia patients and persons that haven't any neuropsychiatric disorder. Nevertheless, the test accuracy is higher than MME, FAST and other tests of dementia.

As a matter of fact, the PAL test is reputed to be able to check the brain area which will be first affected by the disease.

However, early diagnosis is the only alternative for patients to manage the condition because dementia can't be treated as of now!

Specifically, Dementia stats show that 20% of people over 85 years and 2% to 5% of people over 65 years are suffering from dementia. But, early diagnosis and detection remains an essential factor for treating dementia effectively.

Nevertheless, there are many other diagnoses and screenings that are used to eliminate possible causes of memory loss.

And fortunately, there are drug therapies that can slow down the progression of this frightening disease as well!

Dementia! – The Diet Plan Solution

Dementia is a medical word or terminology used to define various symptoms of cognitive deterioration such as forgetfulness which diminishes a person's ability to perform his or her everyday activities as earlier explained in the previous chapter.

Yes, people who are diagnosed with dementia suffer faster decline in mental ability than a person would have due to aging.

Types of Dementia:

The most common type of dementia is Alzheimer's disease, which make about 50% to 70% of the diagnosis of all dementia cases. Other common types include vascular dementia, Lewy body dementia and syphilis.

Symptoms You Can Watch Out For:

Symptoms of dementia are found to be varying among peoples of different age groups and otherwise.

But the most common of them include memory distortions, speech and language difficulty and trouble eating and swallowing. Other symptoms include anxiety, depression, delusions and changes in sleep pattern.

Although, Dementia is incurable, however, by keeping a healthy and balanced diet, you can delay its onset a little longer. It's a scientific fact that as we age and grow older our mind keeps getting weaker and tends to become slow.

But to avoid this medical condition at the early stage of our lives, scientist and researchers recommend diets that can reduce the risks of dementia and Alzheimer.

Dementia Diet And Nutrition…What Works Against Dementia!

Antioxidants such as vitamin-A, beta-carotene and vitamin C and E all are found low in people with Alzheimer's disease.

So, it is concluded that a lot of antioxidants will help you maintain a strong, sharp memory and healthy brain.

Apart from antioxidants, Omega-3 fats, which is found mostly in carnivores, cold water fish such as salmon, tuna and herring also reduces your risk of being diagnosed with dementia and Alzheimer's disease by 60%.

No doubt, a healthy dementia diet will surely keep you away from these diseases but, we can't rely solely on diet.

So, remaining stress free with a relaxed brain is equally crucial such that your brain can function more efficiently and for a prolonged period of time.

In addition to vitamins and omega-3 fats, fruits are something that we should all eat to stay healthy and protected not only from dementia and Alzheimer's disease but from many other diseases as well.

Indeed, Dementia diet control will surely benefit your staying healthy especially when combined with playing some games, which involve mind training such as chess and other games where the memory is extensively used. Yes, this can really be profitable.

In addition, a good mind exercise is like a healthy food for the brain. And if the brain is healthy, then there are less chances of getting diagnosed with Dementia or Alzheimer's disease.

Also, insulin and blood sugar level affects your brain as well as your memory. Do not forget to keep track of your blood sugar levels and maintain a consistent level of insulin and blood sugar levels.

Specific food items such as whole grains, berries and cherries, pumpkin, almonds, omega-3, cashews and walnuts can certainly make a difference if you avoid them or take them.

The truth is that food is the only thing we can make use of and a lot of exercising of the mind and body that will certainly benefit us from all such diseases.

Of course, the side effects of aging on our brain can't be controlled by us but more serious and harmful diseases like Alzheimer's disease and other dementia diseases can be controlled by a balanced diet and some other factors already discussed above.

The Difference Between Alzheimer's Disease And Dementia!

A friend once asked me what the difference was between Alzheimer's disease and dementia. At the time, my knowledge of dementia was petite.

In my understanding, the two were the same, but I later realized that my understanding was somewhat true and false at the same time. I know it sounds funny, right? Let me explain...

When you take your time to research on health issues affecting the elderly, you won't get very far before coming across Alzheimer's disease and dementia.

While they are commonly mentioned together, it is not always clear what the relationship between dementia and Alzheimer's disease really is.

Below is a discussion of dementia and how it relates to Alzheimer's disease as well as some information on other forms of non-Alzheimer's diseases summarized from past reports on Alzheimer's disease from respected health associations:

So, what's the difference between Alzheimer's disease and Dementia?

Well, for starters, Dementia and Alzheimer's disease are not the same things, and that's why they are often spoken of as two different diseases.

The fact is that the term dementia is a generalized term describing multiple forms of diseases that destroy a person's brain neurons and result in diminished intellectual capacity.

Dementia is a general term for these diseases, Alzheimer's disease on the other hand, is the most common and well-known form of dementia.

Alzheimer's disease differs from other types of dementia in the manner in which it attacks the brain. Specifically, the damage results from deposits of proteins in the vascular system of the brain resulting in neuron death.

There are two proteins involved. The first is a protein called "tau". Strands of tau become twisted, and deposit as plaques (the other form of plaque take the form of fragments of the protein beta-amyloid.)

Below are a few common cognitive symptoms of the disease.

The symptoms include; withdrawal from work and/or social activities, disruption of daily life routines owing to severe memory loss, misplacing items and increased disability in retracing steps.

Besides, there is also reduced capacity in planning and solving problems, confusion with time or place, mood or personality changes become noticeable, decreased or poor judgments, increase difficulty with familiar tasks at home or work, development of problems with speaking or writing words etc.

Alzheimer's disease gets the bulk of attention when discussing dementia as it should. However, there are other forms of dementia as well. The next most common to be seen in senior citizens is vascular dementia.

In this form of the disease, symptoms are often very similar to Alzheimer's disease including memory loss; however, the level of memory loss is typically not as severe.

But, damage from vascular dementia comes from arterial blockages resulting from multiple small strokes. The accumulation of impairment reduces blood flow to the brain resulting in neuron death.

The next most common form of dementia is called mixed dementia, and as you might have guessed, it is a disease that results from impairment from multiple types of brain damage.

Typically, the two most common forms of damage stem from the effects of Alzheimer's disease and vascular destruction. But mixed dementia is certainly not limited to just these two types.

"Lewy bodies", which is a disease resulting from the abnormal accumulation of the protein alpha-synuclein in nerve cells of the brain is seen as well. Mixed dementia is being recognized as a more common form of dementia than previously believed.

However, there are so much more underlying causes of dementia that we can discuss, but these other types are becoming rare with time.

Though, the point here is that Alzheimer's disease is basically a form of dementia, not a separate disease. And since it is the most common form, it is the most important to understand.

Understanding Early Signs Of Dementia.

Is it true that most of us are worried about the wellbeing of our old ones or guardians? The fact is that at the point when your folks get more established, you can't make certain that they are dealing with themselves effectively and staying safe.

By and large, your aging parents or guardians may have been seen not to be able to recall certain things for quite a while.

Naturally, in many cases, they will respond by changing the theme of discovering some other subject to supplant the ones they can't discover, while in other scenario, they may stop amidst a sentence or simply work at concealing circumstance!

As a matter of fact, as indicated by a recent study, unmistakably, there are more numbers of aging people who are confronting persistent memory loss and getting rather fed up with life.

The Most Common Early Signs Of Dementia That Can Be Looked For:

Well, to start with, you can check whether they have issues dealing with themselves: - Yes, and most importantly, you ought to give careful consideration to the general appearance of your folks. I mean like, do they look fatigued?

Do they deal with all their day to day routines… undertakings (washing, tooth brushing and other important prep)?

Be that as it may, the truth is that issues with these day to day living activities can without doubt demonstrate, or should I say, display the start of dementia, sorrow or physical hindrances.

Does your dad or mom encounter any memory trouble? : - Yes, it is known that people forget things or overlook things every now and then. But, the fact remains that a reasonable and indeed regular piece of the impact of aging is memory loss!

Without a doubt, every now and then, it has been found as a symptom from the medical condition or it might also be brought on by any underlying condition.

Another thing you might want to consider is, do their memory changes make them to lose things or once in a while forget their name or birth date?

On the other hand, these memory changes are more obvious like neglecting to complete a sentence, getting lost while driving or confronting difficulties to take after straightforward headings.

However, if you are highly worried about the memory loss of your aging parents, you ought to reach for what the human services office have to offer.

Do your aging parents feel safe in their own home? : - Yes, you need to review the encompassing environment of your guardian's/parent's home especially in Ocean County and check whether any of the regions can be a potential danger for them.

Do your folks have difficulty getting to specific segments of their home? : Again, it may look simple and safe to say that they are having issues exploring the stairs?

But at that point, you need to realize, it is time you have to pick up a home human service administration, who offers help with everyday living to guarantee a sheltered and sound environment for them.

Do Your Aging Parents Lose Weight? : - Yes, without doubt, reliable weight reduction can be an early indication of wellbeing issues in aging people.

However, there are so many variables that can add to their undesirable weight reduction. So, you need to check and be sure to know what next to do. The variables among others are:

- They may be challenged with difficulty in getting dinners ready.
- They could be having dexterity issues, getting a handle on cooking utensils or taking after subtle formula elements and additionally perusing labels on food items.
- Losing taste and confronting issues in tasting or swallowing. That is to say, your dad or mom won't be keen on eating if food does not taste or feel great.

Well, by and large, and in fact, all the more regularly, weight reduction could display or should I say is an indication of genuine condition like lack of healthy nutrition, dementia, sadness or growth!

However, if you are worried about the weight reduction of your old ones, then you ought to contact proficient home medicinal services administrations. They usually will have some helping hand to handle the issue and give you some comfort.

Know The Overall Disposition Of Your Parents: - A definitely different point of view can be an early indication of gloominess or other health issues.

Yes, you need to study your old ones' daily routines and particularly, their day to day exercises and social life. Indeed, you need to know whether they visit or connect with friends or not.

I mean, do they have any enthusiasm for their day to day hobbies and other routine exercises? In other words, is it safe to say that they are still connected with clubs, associations or other acquaintances?

In any case, it is important that you know in addition that sadness can be dealt with at any age with specialist intervention.

Just get the assistance of a dependable and reputable home human service organization that can help these old ones to appreciate day to day exercises and other useful activities.

Consequent upon looking through every single early signs of dementia, it's equally recommended to consider essential assistance from home medicinal service and their benefits so that they can help your folks or friends and family keep up their lifestyles and freedom flawlessly.

All You Need to Know About Vascular Dementia…

With all due respect, I want to say that dealing with dementia can be a very daunting ordeal especially if you are new to it.

That's why it is usually advisable that you learn as much as you can about it so that when it comes, you'll be ready!

Well, I must say that there are several varieties of dementia for which they mostly fall into two main categories: primary dementia and secondary dementia. Primary dementia does not result from any other disease.

However, the secondary dementia is caused by another disease or illness which also leads to dementia-like symptoms.

On the other hand, the two most prevalent kinds of dementia are Alzheimer's disease with 60% of all dementia cases, and Vascular Dementia which accounts for 20%.

Now, without doubt, the cause of Vascular Dementia lies in an obstructed blood supply mainly as a result of a series of small strokes. And usually a sudden onset of symptoms is indicative of this condition.

Yes, because of the very way it occurs, vascular dementia has a severe impact on memory and cognitive functioning. However, early treatment can limit the consequences.

A Few Reasons Why It Is Critical To Seek Medical Attention

The truth is that, sometimes, the symptoms you have are quite similar to those of vascular dementia while the cause is different.

For example, people with stress or more severe burn-out can present symptoms as if they suffer from any kind of dementia.

Nevertheless, with a proper diagnosis, the cause in such cases will be discovered and must be treated, then the symptoms will disappear.

Without question, that's a good reason to take action instead of just waiting to see. Besides that, there are more conditions that should be treated immediately because there are many more types of dementia than only vascular dementia… and in a couple of these cases, some treatments are available.

However, I want to add that, it is always the best thing for you to consult your doctor before applying any medication.

A Few Tips On How To Handle This Disease In Its Early Stages

As I have said before, consult your doctor as soon as possible. Then you can write down all of your symptoms and thoughts about it.

Also, ask your relatives to tell you what strikes them about changes in your behavior.

In addition to this, you can also immediately schedule regular follow-up visits with your doctor to keep a record of the progress of your symptoms.

But, it will be helpful also to read extensively about dementia – yes, vascular dementia to be more particular… it helped me a lot in the past.

There are all kinds of books and also the Internet is a good source for such information. With the right information, you can organize your life in a way to make the optimum of it for as long as possible.

Bear in mind that this type of dementia occurs when the arteries to the brain are blocked, and oxygen is cut off, resulting in the death of some brain cells.

It is most common in individuals who have high blood pressure, high cholesterol, diabetes or people who smoke.

Besides that, there are a couple of reasons and causes due to which vascular dementia can take place. Stroke is another reason due to which a person may get prone to this disease.

However, to treat this problem, though, there are so many medicines available, it is equally true that it is not completely curable!

But, its signs and symptoms can certainly get reduced to the barest minimum when identified and treated appropriately as well as promptly.

Now, in conclusion, you should also know that the brain's emotional memories show more resistance to dementia than factual memories.

As a consequence, you might realize that your loved one seems to be always angry with you for no apparent reason.

This is because individuals with dementia usually forget the situations that instigated their strong feelings, but those feelings remain in them even after the incident.

I remember one time that my dad was furious with me in response to my suggestion to help him do something.

The truth is that, the bitterness lingered in him even when he had already forgotten why he was unhappy with me. However, I later came to discover that he was not in any way trying to mistreat me.

Symptoms Of The Stages Of Dementia

Most people who develop dementia start out by showing a lot of forgetfulness. Since this is a normal part of the aging process, people tend to ignore it in the initial stages. Yes, the truth is that, it is only when the condition worsens that people will start to notice!

But let me be upfront with you here, not every patient will show every symptom, however, the disease progresses in all patients in a similar way.

As a matter of fact, dementia occurs in three stages. The first stage of dementia occurs with the vague memory lapses that may bring memory loss to your attention after a while.

During this time your parent may forget their way back home, a phone number, their routine, financial status, and more.

The second stage of dementia becomes more noticeable with every occurrence. In fact, the second stage of dementia can alter the way they do everyday skills such as simple household chores or cooking.

Yes, simple dressing skills and personal hygiene skills may also be noticed as well. Besides that, some speech problems can also be seen.

The third and final stage of dementia can affect the body physically as well as mentally. In fact, they may experience some physical weakness that affects only one side of the body.

You would begin to observe that the muscle tone deteriorates during this stage of dementia, and it might change how they move around. They may start to make up sentences that do not make any sense!

For a caregiver, it's hard to watch someone go through these stages of dementia because you feel as though you can't do anything about it.

However, when a loved one is suffering from dementia, there are several things that you can do to help them feel comfortable and delay the effects that dementia has.

Therefore, when you first suspect that a loved one is suffering from dementia, you need to contact the doctor as soon as possible so you can work together to help them. Keep reminding them of everyday life and routine.

Be sure to keep pictures around everywhere for reminders to help them refresh their memory on a regular basis. If a loved one lives alone, you may want to talk to them about moving in with family.

Find ways to keep their minds constantly occupied such as puzzles and activities outside of the home with other elderly people.

It's important to realize that every day you spend with them is truly a blessing and don't take it personal when they don't recognize you sometimes.

Also, take time each day to ask them to lend a hand in the kitchen or with outdoor chores that they normally do.

They may not be able to do the entire task by themselves but, going through the process can trigger some memories and help minimize depression. So, allow them to work at their pace.

The Three Distinct Stages Of Dementia Are:

- *Early stage* - Symptoms at this juncture include forgetfulness, apathy, absent-mindedness, loss of interest in taking the initiative in activities, confusion, disorientation, memory loss, personality changes, diminished judgment, sudden mood swings, and irritability.

  Well, without doubt, since these same symptoms can be part of other diseases as well as aging, it's often difficult to diagnose dementia until it progresses to at least the moderate stage.

- *Moderate stage* – Yes, this is the stage where most diagnosis is confirmed… during this juncture symptoms become easier to identify and positively diagnose the condition.

- *Advanced stage* - At this point in the progression of the condition, patients need continuous care. In fact, they no longer speak or communicate in any way at this stage. They show no response to people around them and can no longer recognize family members or everyday objects as usual.

As a matter of fact, some of the severe symptoms that develop at this stage include random movements, incontinence, mobility issues, insomnia, significant memory loss, and the inability to perform simple daily tasks for themselves.

Yes, in this advanced stage, the patient will require a nursing home or an assisted living care.

Though, it's often said that dementia is an incurable sickness of the aging ones… but I dare say that in a few cases, dementia may be reversible if caught and treated early.

Well, in the real sense, I will say for most patients, treatment consists of presenting the patient with activities to help the mind stay sharp, feeding them a nutritious diet, and making them as comfortable as possible. All these will certainly go a long way to help them.

Wrap Up

Thank you for downloading this book!

I hope you enjoyed reading my book on *Vascular Dementia: The Complete Dementia Caregiver's Guide with Tips on Dementia and What You Need to Know to Manage the Condition from the Onset of Dementia Symptoms Today!*

Anyway, if you enjoyed this book, please take the time to share your thoughts and post a review for me. It would be greatly appreciated!

Thank you!

Made in the USA
Coppell, TX
30 January 2021

49124293R10018